How To Lose Weight Without A Diet

The Ultimate Guide to Sustainable Weight Loss and Healthy Living

by Steve Marvell

By sharing a review of this book, wherever you discovered it, you can inspire others to take their first steps towards a healthier, more fulfilling life. Your story, your insights, and your reflections might be the spark that helps someone else embrace positive change. Together, we can create a ripple effect of encouragement and empowerment, helping more people discover the freedom of living healthily without the burden of dieting.

Thank you for being part of this journey and for sharing the gift of better health with others.

CONTENTS

DISCLAIMER

This document, titled "How To Lose Weight Without A Diet" is provided for informational purposes only and is not intended as medical advice, diagnosis, or treatment. The contents of this document are not a substitute for professional medical advice, diagnosis, or treatment. Always seek the advice of your physician or other qualified health provider with any questions you may have regarding a medical condition, diet, fitness, or wellness program.

Before starting any new diet or fitness regimen, it is essential to consult with a healthcare professional, especially if you have any pre-existing health conditions or concerns. The information provided in this document is intended to support, not replace, the relationship between you and your healthcare providers.

The author(s) and publisher(s) of " How To Lose Weight Without A Diet " are not responsible for any adverse effects or consequences resulting from the use of any suggestions, preparations, or methods described in this document. Use of the information in this document is at your own risk.

The nutritional information and guidelines provided in this document may not be suitable for everyone, particularly individuals with specific dietary needs or health concerns. It is important to tailor any diet or fitness program to your individual needs, preferences, and medical conditions.

No guarantee is made regarding the results that may be obtained from following the recommendations in this document. Results vary from person to person, and success in weight management and lifestyle improvement depends on a variety of factors, including individual commitment, health status, and adherence to guidelines.

INTRODUCTION

Effectively losing weight without dieting might sound too good to be true, but that's exactly what this book is about. Forget restrictive meal plans, calorie counting, and the endless cycle of fad diets. Instead, this is your guide to achieving a healthier, happier you through practical, sustainable changes that fit seamlessly into your everyday life. It's about creating a lifestyle that works for you—one that prioritises balance, joy, and long-term success over short-term deprivation.

You'll discover strategies that go beyond the plate, exploring how movement, mindset, habits, and self-awareness play a pivotal role in lasting weight loss. This book dives into how small, consistent tweaks to your routine can lead to big changes over time. It's not about "going on a diet" but about equipping yourself with tools to make better choices, fuel your body, and feel great without feeling restricted.

Throughout, you'll learn how to recognise what your body truly needs, overcome common challenges, and build habits that last a lifetime. From understanding the science behind weight loss to finding joy in movement and nourishment, this book aims to transform the way you think about your health. It's not just about losing weight—it's about gaining confidence, energy, and a sense of balance that empowers you to live your best life.

Health isn't just about a number on the scales or fitting into a smaller size; it's about embracing a mindset that prioritises wellness, balance, and vitality in every aspect of life. For anyone seeking a healthier lifestyle, the journey towards weight loss and improved well-being is an opportunity to reshape not only your body but also your outlook, habits, and confidence. It's a process that can transform your life, challenge you physically and mentally, and set you on a path towards lasting health and happiness.

This journey is about so much more than shedding pounds. It's about embracing a lifestyle that enhances every part of your well-being—physical, emotional, and mental. When you approach weight loss as an opportunity to grow and thrive, rather than as a chore or a punishment, it becomes a powerful and rewarding process. By shifting the focus from restrictive dieting to sustainable, enjoyable habits, you'll find that the changes you make are not only effective but deeply fulfilling.

As you embark on this path, you'll begin to notice the benefits ripple through all aspects of your life. From increased energy and physical resilience to a boost in confidence and emotional health, every small step forward builds toward a more vibrant and capable you. Let's take a closer look at the many ways this journey can transform your life, starting with the physical rewards of improved health and fitness.

Enhanced Physical Well-being

Losing weight improves physical capabilities like endurance, strength, and flexibility. This makes daily activities easier, allowing you to enjoy your favourite pastimes with greater comfort and ease. Even simple actions, like climbing stairs or carrying groceries, become less taxing, and you'll find yourself moving through life with increased physical freedom and resilience.

Boosted Energy Levels

With fewer excess pounds, your body becomes more efficient, allowing for heightened energy throughout the day. This boost helps you maintain focus at work, enjoy active hobbies, and tackle daily tasks with enthusiasm. You'll feel revitalised and ready to make the most of every moment.

Improved Emotional and Mental Health

The journey towards a healthier body often brings profound emotional benefits. Achieving your goals can boost self-esteem and reduce stress, while the structure of healthy habits supports mental clarity and stability. Each milestone along the way reinforces your sense of accomplishment and builds resilience for future challenges.

Holistic Health Benefits

Weight loss contributes to improved overall health, including better cardiovascular function, stronger immunity, and enhanced sleep quality. These changes promote long-term well-being, allowing you to feel your best and reduce the risk of chronic illnesses. The ripple effect of these benefits extends to every area of your life, improving not just your health but your daily experiences.

Sustainable Lifestyle Changes

True weight loss isn't about quick fixes or restrictive diets; it's about creating a sustainable lifestyle. Adopting balanced eating habits that prioritise wholesome, nutritious foods ensures you're nourishing your body while still enjoying occasional indulgences. By finding this balance, you can maintain your results and live a fulfilling life without the constant cycle of dieting.

Embarking on a weight loss journey is about far more than the physical changes—it's an opportunity to rediscover yourself, build confidence, and create a life filled with energy and purpose. Each step forward is a step towards a healthier, more vibrant you, capable of tackling life with enthusiasm and joy.

This is not just a process of transformation; it's an act of self-empowerment. By embracing this journey, you're investing in your health, your future, and your ability to live life fully. The challenges along the way may test your resolve, but the rewards of a healthier body and a more balanced lifestyle make every effort worthwhile.

EMBRACING A HEALTHIER LIFESTYLE WITH SIMPLE CHANGES

Transitioning to a healthier lifestyle and achieving weight loss doesn't mean completely changing your routine or giving up the foods you enjoy. It's about making small, manageable adjustments that seamlessly fit into your daily life while supporting your goals. By focusing on these simple, sustainable changes, you can lose weight naturally and maintain it without restrictive diets. Whether you're balancing a busy schedule, family commitments, or personal projects, these strategies will help you create a lifestyle that promotes weight loss while still embracing the joy of eating and living fully.

Hydrate Adequately

Drinking plenty of water throughout the day might seem simple, but it's a game-changer for your health. Staying hydrated aids digestion, boosts energy, and even curbs unnecessary snacking. But hydration isn't just about quantity—it's about consistency and making water an integral part of your daily habits.

Use Smaller Plates

Using smaller plates might seem like a trivial change, but it's an impactful way to reshape your eating habits. By naturally reducing portion sizes, you can enjoy the satisfaction of a full plate without overindulging. This subtle shift helps you retrain your mind to recognise smaller meals as just as fulfilling as larger ones, paving the way for long-term, sustainable balance.

Eat Mindfully

Mindful eating is a practice that transforms mealtimes into an experience of awareness and enjoyment. It's about tuning into your body's signals, savouring every bite, and appreciating the nourishment your food provides. By slowing down and eliminating distractions, you can better connect with what your body needs and break the cycle of mindless snacking or overeating.

Portion Control

Portion control is less about restriction and more about learning to listen to your body's cues. Starting with smaller servings and giving yourself time to recognise fullness allows you to enjoy your meals without excess. This approach helps you appreciate quality over quantity, creating a sense of satisfaction that supports your goals without feeling deprived.

Store Leftovers Wisely

Leftovers aren't just a convenience; they're an opportunity to stay on track with your health goals. By storing and repurposing meals creatively, you can save time, reduce waste, and always have nutritious options on hand. With a little planning, yesterday's dinner can become today's quick, balanced solution, keeping your routine both practical and rewarding.

Avoid Food as a Reward

Rewarding yourself with food might feel comforting in the moment, but it can tie emotions to eating in ways that are hard to break. Instead, finding joy in other celebrations—like new experiences or personal achievements—can create a more positive relationship with both food and yourself. This shift allows you to focus on what truly fulfils you, without using food as the focal point.

Shop on a Full Stomach

Shopping when you're hungry is a recipe for impulsive decisions and less-than-healthy purchases. By heading to the store after a meal or snack, you'll find it easier to stick to your list and focus on foods that truly nourish you. This simple habit transforms your shopping trips into opportunities to support your long-term goals without distractions.

Keep a Healthy Kitchen

Your kitchen sets the tone for your eating habits, and keeping it stocked with wholesome, nourishing options makes healthy choices effortless. By creating an environment where nutritious foods are within easy reach, you can remove temptation and foster a lifestyle that supports balance, variety, and satisfaction.

Focus on Fit, Not Weight

Numbers on a scale tell only part of the story, but how your clothes fit can reveal so much more. Shifting your focus to how you feel in your body—stronger, more flexible, more energetic—helps you celebrate progress in meaningful ways. This approach prioritises well-being over perfection, creating a healthier, more positive mindset.

Prioritise Sleep

Sleep is one of the most overlooked foundations of good health, yet it's critical for managing weight, energy, and mood. Restorative sleep keeps your hormones balanced, your cravings in check, and your body functioning at its best. By giving sleep the importance it deserves, you're laying the groundwork for success in every aspect of your well-being.

Invest in a Healthy Cookbook

A cookbook filled with quick, nutritious recipes can be your secret weapon for maintaining variety and excitement in your meals. It inspires creativity, introduces new flavours, and simplifies the process of preparing balanced dishes that fit into your busy life. With the right resources, healthy eating becomes a joy rather than a chore.

These tips are designed to fit seamlessly into busy, active lives, helping you adopt simple, effective strategies for a balanced and sustainable approach to eating. This is key to achieving long-term health and wellness goals by fostering lasting habits rather than temporary fixes. When your choices support your energy and well-being, maintaining a fulfilling lifestyle becomes much easier. Embracing these changes enhances your physical health and enriches every aspect of your life, allowing you to move forward with vitality and confidence.

HYDRATE ADEQUATELY
DRINK PLENTY OF WATER

Hydration is a cornerstone of good health, influencing every aspect of bodily function. It plays a crucial role in weight management, physical performance, and overall well-being, especially if you value staying active. Understanding the importance of proper hydration can significantly enhance your health journey. Here's an in-depth look at why staying hydrated is essential:

Appetite Control and Weight Management

Thirst is often mistaken for hunger, leading to unnecessary calorie consumption. By staying well-hydrated, you can better distinguish between hunger and thirst cues, preventing overeating. Drinking a glass of water before meals can create a sense of fullness, potentially reducing your overall calorie intake. This simple habit supports weight management by helping you eat only when genuinely hungry.

Enhanced Metabolic Function

Water is fundamental to the body's metabolic processes. Adequate hydration can slightly boost your metabolic rate, meaning you burn more calories even at rest. This metabolic enhancement supports weight loss efforts and overall energy levels. Additionally, water assists in the transport of nutrients and oxygen to cells, optimizing bodily functions and energy production.

Improved Physical Performance and Endurance

Whether your day includes exercise, work, or play, hydration is key to maintaining peak performance. Even mild dehydration can impair abilities, leading to fatigue, muscle cramps, and decreased motivation. Proper hydration ensures that your muscles are well-nourished and that joint lubrication is optimal, reducing the risk of injuries during physical activities.

Cognitive Function and Mood Regulation

Dehydration doesn't just affect the body; it impacts the mind as well. Insufficient water intake can lead to difficulties in concentration, alertness, and short-term memory. It may also influence mood, causing irritability or feelings of anxiety. By staying hydrated, you support brain function, which is essential for decision-making and fully enjoying your day.

Detoxification and Digestive Health

Water plays a vital role in flushing toxins out of the body through urine and sweat. Adequate hydration supports kidney function, helping to prevent kidney stones and urinary tract infections. In terms of digestion, water aids in breaking down food so that your body can absorb nutrients effectively. Proper hydration helps prevent constipation by keeping the digestive tract moving smoothly.

Healthy Skin and Appearance

Skin is the body's largest organ, and water is essential for maintaining its health and elasticity. Adequate hydration can improve skin complexion, giving it a more vibrant look. This not only boosts confidence but also enhances protection against environmental factors.

Joint Health and Muscle Recovery

Water is a component of synovial fluid, which lubricates and cushions joints. Staying hydrated reduces joint pain and the risk of injury. For muscle recovery, hydration helps in repairing muscle fibres and reducing inflammation after physical exertion.

Regulation of Body Temperature

Especially important during any form of exercise or hot weather, water helps regulate body temperature through sweating. Proper hydration ensures that your body can cool itself efficiently.

How to Hydrate Effectively

1. Set a Daily Water Goal

   Aim for at least 8-10 glasses of water a day. Adjust if you're very active, live in a hot environment, or spend time at high altitudes.

2. Incorporate Hydrating Foods

   Include water-rich foods like cucumbers, watermelon, oranges, strawberries, and lettuce. These also provide essential vitamins and minerals.

3. Monitor Urine Colour

   Pale yellow indicates proper hydration, while darker shades suggest you need more fluids.

4. Limit Dehydrating Beverages

   Be mindful of diuretics like alcohol and caffeinated drinks, which can increase fluid loss. Balance these with adequate water.

5. Carry a Reusable Water Bottle

   Having water available encourages regular sipping throughout the day.

6. Set Reminders

   Use phone alarms or apps to remind you to drink water regularly, especially if you tend to forget when busy.

7. Listen to Your Body

   Thirst is a late indicator of dehydration. Try to drink water consistently before you feel thirsty.

By making water intake a priority, you support your body's natural processes and contribute significantly to your overall health and weight management goals. Staying hydrated enhances physical performance, cognitive function, and mood, all of which are crucial for living life to the fullest. Embracing proper hydration is a simple yet powerful step toward a healthier, more vibrant life.

USE SMALLER PLATES
CONTROL PORTIONS EFFORTLESSLY

Using smaller plates is a simple yet effective strategy for managing portion sizes and reducing overall calorie intake. This approach relies on visual cues and can seamlessly fit into a balanced lifestyle. Here's how it works and why it's beneficial:

Visual Illusion and Perception

A phenomenon called the Delboeuf illusion shows that the same amount of food appears larger on a smaller plate than on a larger one. This tricks your brain into feeling satisfied with less food. When your plate looks full, your mind registers it as a complete meal, which can reduce the likelihood of going back for seconds.

Automatic Portion Control Without Effort

Smaller plates naturally limit how much food you serve yourself, helping to prevent overeating. It's a form of portion control that doesn't require calorie counting or constant measuring. Over time, this leads to a reduction in daily calorie consumption, supporting weight management goals.

Promotes Mindful Eating Habits

A full smaller plate signals that you're consuming a satisfying portion. This can encourage you to eat more slowly and savour each bite—core principles of mindful eating. By being fully present, you're more likely to recognize fullness cues and avoid overeating.

Adaptable to Any Cuisine and Dining Environment

Whether you're at home, dining out, at a social gathering, or traveling, choosing a smaller plate is a subtle shift that doesn't feel restrictive. It allows you to enjoy diverse cuisines while still keeping portions in check.

Easy to Implement with Immediate Impact

Switching to smaller plates requires minimal effort but can significantly affect your eating habits. It feels less like a diet and more like a gentle boundary, making it easier to stick to in the long run.

Reduces Food Waste and Encourages Sustainability

By serving smaller portions, you're less likely to leave food uneaten on your plate, reducing waste. This practice aligns with a mindful and responsible lifestyle.

Enhances Dining Experience and Satisfaction

Smaller plates can make meals feel more indulgent because they appear abundant. This visual fullness enhances the overall dining experience and reinforces positive associations with healthy eating.

Supports a Lifestyle of Simplicity and Mindfulness

This approach blends well with a simpler, more intentional way of living. By streamlining portion control, you free up mental energy for other important life pursuits.

Encourages Family and Social Health Habits

The use of smaller plates can influence those around you to adopt similar habits, fostering a supportive environment for healthier eating. It also pairs well with other strategies like incorporating more vegetables or focusing on whole foods.

Combines Well with Other Healthy Eating Strategies

Smaller plates complement approaches like mindful eating, balanced meal composition, and portion awareness, making it a flexible tool regardless of dietary preferences.

Why Plate Size is So Effective?

Imagine you're using a **large plate** with a diameter of 30 cm (12 inches). Typically, plates have a border of about 2.5 cm (1 inch) where no food is placed, leaving a usable area of around 25 cm (10 inches) in diameter for food.

Now compare that to a **standard smaller plate** with a diameter of 23 cm (9 inches). With the same 2.5 cm (1 inch) border, the usable area shrinks to about 18 cm (7 inches) in diameter.

That three-inch reduction does not take a third off the portion; it actually reduces the usable area by nearly 50%. This is because the area of a circle increases exponentially with its diameter. A large plate with a 25 cm (10 inches) usable area has almost twice the space of a smaller plate with an 18 cm (7 inches) usable area. Even though the plates might not look drastically different at first glance, the smaller plate encourages significantly smaller portions, helping you cut down on how much you serve without even realising it.

What's even more fascinating is how this impacts your perception of satisfaction. When you fill a smaller plate, it looks visually abundant—there's no empty space, and the food appears generous. On a larger plate, the same amount of food can look sparse and inadequate, leading you to add more to compensate. This visual illusion is powerful: your brain associates a full plate with a satisfying meal, regardless of the actual quantity. By using a smaller plate, you're not just eating less—you're also tricking your mind into feeling just as content as you would with a larger serving. This subtle psychological shift allows you to embrace smaller portions without feeling deprived, making it easier to maintain healthier eating habits over time.

Shopping List for Crockery and Cutlery

Here is a practical shopping list with recommended sizes for smaller crockery to help with portion control. The sizes are listed in centimetres first, followed by inches in parentheses.

Plates

1. Side Plates (for main meals): 20–23 cm (8–9 inches) diameter

   Smaller than the standard dinner plate (26–28 cm / 10–11 inches) but large enough for a balanced meal.

2. Dessert Plates (for light meals or snacks): 15–18 cm (6–7 inches) diameter

   Perfect for smaller portions or for visually "filling" the plate.

Bowls

3. Cereal/Salad Bowls: 12–15 cm (5–6 inches) diameter, 6–8 cm (2.5–3 inches) deep

   Ideal for portioning soups, cereals, or salads without overloading.

4. Snack or Dessert Bowls: 10–12 cm (4–5 inches) diameter, 5–6 cm (2–2.5 inches) deep

   Great for small servings of yoghurt, fruits, or desserts.

Cups and Glasses

5. Mugs: 200–250 ml capacity (7–9 fl oz)

   Slightly smaller than standard mugs (300–350 ml / 10–12 fl oz) to help with portion control for beverages like coffee or tea.

6. Juice Glasses: 150–200 ml capacity (5–7 fl oz)

A smaller option for portioning juices or other calorie-dense drinks.

Serving Dishes

7. Small Serving Bowls: 18–20 cm (7–8 inches) diameter

Helps manage portion sizes when serving dishes family-style.

8. Platter for Shared Dishes: 25 cm (10 inches) length

Compact yet functional for serving shared appetisers or small portions of sides.

Cutlery (Optional for Smaller Portions)

9. Dessert Forks and Spoons: 16–18 cm (6–7 inches) length

Smaller than standard forks/spoons (20 cm / 8 inches), promoting smaller bites.

By choosing crockery that aligns with these dimensions, you can subtly reduce portion sizes without feeling restricted, making your meals feel satisfying and balanced.

Select designs, colours, or patterns you genuinely like, as this can make the process more enjoyable and turn each meal into a more positive and engaging experience. When your plates are something you look forward to using, it reinforces your commitment to this change, making it easier to maintain over time.

Incorporating smaller plates into your routine is an easy, practical way to manage portions without feeling deprived. It aligns with a mindset that values simplicity and mindfulness, ultimately helping you reach and maintain your health goals while fully enjoying your meals.

EAT MINDFULLY
LISTEN TO YOUR BODY'S HUNGER CUES

Mindful eating offers a wide range of benefits that extend beyond portion control. By bringing attention to the act of eating, you not only transform your relationship with food but also enjoy positive impacts on your physical, emotional, and mental well-being. Here are some key benefits of incorporating mindful eating into your life:

Improved Digestion

Mindful eating involves chewing food thoroughly and eating at a slower pace. This helps your digestive system break down food more efficiently, reducing discomforts like bloating, indigestion, or heartburn. By allowing your body time to process each bite, you give it the best chance to absorb nutrients effectively.

Reduced Cravings

When you tune into your hunger cues, you can better distinguish between true physical hunger and cravings driven by emotions or habits. This awareness makes it easier to resist the pull of sugary, salty, or processed foods.

Enhanced Emotional Well-Being

Eating mindfully introduces calmness to your meals, transforming them into moments of self-care. This practice reduces stress, promotes relaxation, and creates a sense of control, helping you feel emotionally grounded even on busy or challenging days.

Greater Food Appreciation

When you take time to savour your meals, you build a deeper connection to the food on your plate. This fosters gratitude for the effort and resources that go into nourishing yourself, which can inspire healthier choices and reduce reliance on convenience foods.

Increased Satisfaction

The sensory focus of mindful eating allows you to fully enjoy the flavours, textures, and aromas of your food. This heightened awareness makes smaller portions feel just as satisfying as larger ones, supporting long-term healthy habits.

Supports Balanced Eating Patterns

Mindful eating encourages you to respond to your body's needs rather than external cues, such as stress, boredom, or mealtime routines. This adaptability helps you maintain a flexible and balanced approach to food, without guilt or rigidity.

How to Eat Mindfully

1. Eliminate Distractions

   Multitasking during meals—whether watching TV, working, or scrolling on your phone—disconnects you from the act of eating. A calm, dedicated eating environment allows you to focus on your meal and your body's internal signals. By removing distractions, you'll find it easier to control portions and experience greater satisfaction.

2. Understand Hunger Cues

   Recognising true hunger is the first step toward mindful eating. Physical hunger develops gradually and can be satisfied by various foods, often presenting as a growling stomach or low energy. Emotional hunger, on the other hand, tends to come on suddenly and is linked to cravings for specific comfort foods. By pausing to assess whether you're truly hungry or simply eating in response to emotions, you can prevent unnecessary calorie intake and create a healthier relationship with food.

3. Chew Thoroughly

   Proper chewing isn't just about digestion—it's about slowing down and enjoying your food. Take time to notice the taste and texture of each bite, aiming to chew thoroughly before swallowing. This practice aids in digestion, reduces overeating, and enhances your overall dining experience.

4. Savour Your Food

   Focus on the flavours, textures, aromas, and presentation of your meals. This heightened awareness enhances your enjoyment and can leave you feeling more content with smaller portions. Additionally, noticing what satisfies you most can guide you toward more nourishing and fulfilling food choices.

5. Check-In Mid-Meal

Pausing halfway through your meal to assess your hunger level is a simple yet effective way to practice mindfulness. This short pause allows you to decide whether you truly need more or have had enough.

6. Recognize Fullness

Paying attention to fullness cues is just as important. Eating slowly allows you to notice when you're comfortably satisfied rather than uncomfortably full. It takes about 20 minutes for your brain to register satiety, so slowing your pace can prevent overeating. Try placing your cutlery down between bites or pausing mid-meal to reflect on whether you still feel hungry.

7. Be Aware of Emotional Eating

Stress, boredom, loneliness, and even happiness can trigger cravings for comfort foods. Becoming aware of these emotional drivers is essential. Instead of turning to food, develop healthier coping strategies like going for a walk, practising relaxation techniques, or engaging in a creative hobby. Mindful awareness of these triggers helps you respond more constructively.

Mindful eating is about how you eat, not just what you eat. By cultivating this awareness, you'll become more in tune with your body's signals, leading to wiser food choices and greater satisfaction. With practice, it supports long-term weight management, reduces stress often linked to dieting, and makes meals more enjoyable overall. Use this as an opportunity to reconnect with food, your body, and the act of eating in a way that empowers you.

TAKE SMALLER PORTIONS AND COME BACK FOR SECONDS IF NEEDED

Choosing smaller portions initially—with the freedom to grab more if you're still hungry—is an effective strategy for controlling food intake while respecting your hunger signals. This approach aligns with a lifestyle that values balance and mindfulness:

Prevents Overeating

Starting with smaller portions naturally reduces how much you eat, as you're less likely to overfill your plate or feel pressured to clear it. By taking only what you need initially, you avoid the guilt of leaving food uneaten or wasting it. This simple habit allows you to enjoy your meal without overindulging.

Encourages Mindful Eating

Pausing to decide on seconds prompts you to ask if you're genuinely hungry or just eating out of habit. This pause promotes mindfulness and can reduce mindless overeating.

Increases Portion Size Awareness

Frequently checking your hunger and the amount of food you consume refines your understanding of portions. This helps avoid unintentionally oversized servings, especially when confronted with large plates or buffet-style meals.

Supports Gradual Change

For anyone used to large servings, this approach offers a gentle transition. It avoids drastic alterations that can feel restrictive or overwhelming, making sustainable eating changes more achievable. Instead of focusing on what you're cutting back, this method reframes smaller portions as a way to savour your meal and feel more in control.

Reduces Food Waste

Smaller initial servings mean less chance of leftovers that get thrown away, which lowers waste and aligns with a more eco-conscious approach. If you do have leftovers, they can be easily stored and repurposed for another meal. This not only reduces waste but also saves time and money, reinforcing the practicality of this method.

This habit balances flexibility and mindfulness, letting you enjoy meals without unnecessary restrictions while still supporting healthier portion sizes. Over time, it fosters self-awareness, discipline, and a more satisfying relationship with food.

STORE LEFTOVERS WISELY
FREEZE OR REPURPOSE THE FUTURE

Properly handling leftovers is economical and ensures you always have healthy options on hand, which is especially important for those with busy routines. Here's how to optimize your leftovers:

Healthy Convenience

Leftovers offer a quick and hassle-free way to stay on track with healthy eating, especially on busy days when time is limited. Instead of resorting to processed or fast food, having a variety of pre-prepared, nutritious options in your fridge or freezer ensures that you always have a wholesome meal at your fingertips. For instance, a leftover portion of roasted vegetables and grains can easily become a satisfying lunch bowl with a drizzle of dressing. Knowing that healthy meals are ready to go eliminates decision fatigue and makes maintaining a balanced diet effortless, even during hectic schedules.

Reduced Food Waste

Leftovers play a significant role in cutting food waste by ensuring every ingredient you purchase is fully utilised. Rather than discarding uneaten portions, you can repurpose them into new dishes or save them for later. This eco-friendly habit supports a sustainable lifestyle by reducing the resources needed to produce and transport food. For example, turning leftover mashed potatoes into a topping for shepherd's pie creates a delicious meal while promoting resourcefulness.

Economic Savings

Making the most of leftovers reduces grocery expenses and allows you to stretch your budget further. The money saved can be used for other priorities, such as hobbies or family activities. Leftovers also maximise the value of your meals, ensuring nothing goes to waste. For instance, leftover roast chicken can easily be turned into sandwiches or a hearty soup, helping your shopping budget go further without sacrificing variety or quality.

Enhanced Culinary Creativity

Leftovers inspire creativity in the kitchen, encouraging you to experiment with new recipes and flavour combinations. Transforming ingredients into entirely new dishes prevents boredom and keeps meals interesting. For example, roasted vegetables can become a creamy soup, a frittata filling, or a pasta topping. This experimentation expands your cooking skills and makes meal prep more rewarding and enjoyable.

Less Stress and Time Investment

Having leftovers on hand simplifies daily life by reducing the pressure to cook from scratch every day. Instead of preparing an entire meal, you can reheat or repurpose leftovers, saving time for leisure or family activities. This approach creates a relaxed kitchen environment, helping you maintain a balanced and fulfilling routine.

Strategies for Optimising Leftovers

1. Freeze for Later

    Many dishes, such as soups, casseroles, and stews, freeze well and can be reheated for quick, healthy meals. Use airtight containers or freezer bags and label them with contents and dates. This keeps your freezer stocked with ready-to-eat options for those hectic days.

2. Repurpose Creatively

    Leftovers can be transformed into entirely new dishes to keep meals exciting. For example: Roasted vegetables can become the base for a warming soup or a filling for wraps. Grilled chicken can be shredded into salads, sandwiches, or stir-fries. Cooked rice can be reinvented into a flavourful fried rice or added to grain bowls.

3. Plan for Leftovers

    When cooking, intentionally prepare extra portions. For example, double the amount of roasted vegetables or make additional servings of soup. This ensures you have convenient meals for the next day and reduces the time spent in the kitchen later.

4. Use Leftovers for Healthy Snacking

    Smaller portions of leftovers are perfect as nutritious snacks. Items like roasted chicken, cooked vegetables, or grains provide a wholesome and satisfying alternative to processed snacks, helping you stay energised between meals.

5. Practice Safe Storage

    Store leftovers in airtight containers to preserve freshness and prevent contamination. Label them clearly with contents and dates to ensure timely use. Refrigerated leftovers should be consumed within a few days, while frozen options can be kept for longer.

Consult FSA, NHS, FDA, and FSIS sources for absolute guidance on storage and reuse.

Bubble and Squeak

Bubble and squeak is a classic British dish that transforms leftover vegetables (and sometimes meat) from a previous meal into a hearty and satisfying dish. Traditionally fried, it can be just as delicious when baked or cooked in a non-stick pan with minimal oil, offering a lighter alternative. This simple recipe reduces waste while delivering a comforting meal that's full of flavour.

Ingredients: Equal parts cooked vegetables and potatoes

Preparation: Mash everything together and season

Non-stick pan method: Heat a non-stick pan over medium heat. Add a teaspoon of oil or a light spray of cooking oil. Cook the patties for 3–4 minutes on each side, until golden and heated through.

Oven-baked method: Preheat the oven to 200°C (180°C fan/gas mark 6). Spread the mixture evenly in a lightly greased ovenproof dish. Bake for 20–25 minutes until golden on top and warmed through.

Serving suggestion: Poached Egg and HP Sauce

By weaving leftover management into your meal planning, you conserve both time and money, while consistently having nutritious meals at your fingertips. This method suits busy lifestyles and promotes a balanced, sustainable approach to eating.

AVOID FOOD AS A REWARD
FIND NON-FOOD WAYS TO CELEBRATE

Using food as a reward can disrupt your relationship with eating, tying it to emotions rather than genuine physical hunger. This habit often reinforces patterns of turning to food for comfort, celebration, or stress relief, rather than nourishment. Shifting away from this dynamic is essential for fostering a healthier, more balanced approach to both food and emotional well-being. By exploring alternatives, you can break this cycle and discover more fulfilling ways to celebrate achievements and navigate challenges.

Breaking the Food-Emotion Link

Using food as a reward creates a strong connection between eating and emotional cues rather than genuine physical hunger. This often results in reaching for treats to cope with stress, boredom, or even as a celebration, which can perpetuate unhealthy eating patterns. By avoiding this habit, you foster a more balanced relationship with food, allowing it to return to its true purpose—nourishing your body.

Supporting Long-Term Health

Shifting away from food rewards can significantly benefit your overall health. Calorie-dense, sugary, or fatty foods are commonly used as rewards but often conflict with health and weight goals. By replacing them with non-food alternatives, you align your actions with your long-term objectives and avoid the guilt or regret that often follows indulgence.

Encouraging Personal Growth

Non-food rewards open doors to new opportunities for joy and achievement. Whether it's learning a new skill, engaging in a favourite activity, or exploring a creative passion, these rewards provide a deeper sense of satisfaction. They foster growth, build confidence, and often leave lasting, meaningful memories—something a fleeting treat can't offer.

Strengthening Healthy Eating Habits

As food is no longer tied to emotional triggers, it becomes easier to focus on your body's natural hunger and fullness cues. This separation allows you to make intentional, mindful eating choices that align with your well-being. Over time, these habits become second nature, supporting your physical and emotional health.

Enhancing Emotional Resilience

Choosing non-food rewards encourages you to find healthier ways to celebrate achievements or manage stress. This builds emotional resilience by fostering activities that contribute to a sense of balance and fulfilment, creating a strong foundation for your overall well-being.

How to Reward Yourself Well

1. Identify Meaningful Rewards

    Choose rewards that genuinely excite or inspire you. These might include engaging in a creative hobby, enjoying a spa day, or spending time outdoors. For example, reading a book you've been eager to start or setting aside time for a peaceful walk can provide joy and fulfilment without linking achievements to food.

2. Create a Reward System

    Tracking your goals and assigning rewards can make progress fun and tangible. For instance, after completing a fitness milestone or sticking to a new habit, treat yourself to an enriching experience like a workshop or a relaxing day out. Keeping a visible record of your achievements helps reinforce positive behaviours and adds an element of excitement to your journey.

3. Use Physical Activity as a Reward

    Activities like a yoga session, a scenic hike, or even trying a new fitness class can be highly rewarding. Not only do they celebrate your progress, but they also contribute to your health and energy levels, making them a double win.

4. Invest in Experiences

    Plan experiences that create lasting memories, such as visiting a cultural event, attending a concert, or exploring a new destination. These rewards offer a sense of accomplishment and leave you with something meaningful to reflect on, making them more fulfilling than a temporary indulgence.

5. Prioritise Self-Care

    Pampering yourself can be a reward in itself. Schedule a massage, take a long bath, or enjoy a quiet evening with a favourite film. These moments of relaxation not only help you recharge but also reinforce the value of caring for yourself.

6. Share Your Success

    Celebrating milestones publicly, whether with friends or online, can amplify your sense of accomplishment. Positive feedback and encouragement from others can motivate you to keep progressing, creating a sense of community and shared pride in your achievements.

7. Explore New Skills

    Learning something new can be both rewarding and inspiring. Whether it's picking up a musical instrument, trying a creative craft, or taking a cooking class, these activities provide lasting benefits that extend far beyond the initial reward.

Recognise Emotional Triggers

Understanding why you reach for food can help you break the habit. Reflect on whether stress, boredom, or loneliness is driving your desire for a treat. Once you're aware of these triggers, you can redirect your energy toward healthier coping mechanisms like journaling, deep breathing, or physical activity. These practices not only help in the moment but also cultivate long-term emotional resilience.

By shifting the focus away from food as a reward, you're not only fostering a healthier relationship with eating but also opening the door to new experiences and ways to celebrate life's milestones. This change empowers you to embrace meaningful, lasting rewards that align with your values and goals, supporting both your emotional well-being and physical health. Over time, these choices become habits, reinforcing a balanced, fulfilling lifestyle where food is no longer tied to emotions but cherished as nourishment for body and mind.

SHOP ON A FULL STOMACH
AVOID IMPULSE BUYS

Going grocery shopping when you're hungry often leads to impulsive and less nutritious purchases. Shopping after eating helps you make better decisions, stay on track with your health goals, and even save money.

Reduced Cravings

Hunger makes it harder to resist sugary or high-fat snacks, leading to unhealthy choices. Shopping on a full stomach reduces these temptations, helping you focus on balanced, nourishing foods that support your goals.

Improved Decision-Making

Shopping while hungry often results in impulse buys that don't align with your plans. Eating beforehand helps you stick to your list and make thoughtful choices that support a sustainable and healthy routine.

Budget-Friendly Choices

Impulse buys are often expensive and unnecessary. Shopping after eating helps you avoid overspending and focus on affordable, quality ingredients that fit your budget and health priorities.

Implementing This Strategy

1. Eat a Balanced Meal Before Shopping

    Include protein, fibre, and healthy fats.

2. Schedule Shopping Trips Wisely

    Go after breakfast or lunch to leverage natural satiety.

3. Stay Hydrated

    Thirst can sometimes mimic hunger, so sip water throughout.

4. Avoid Shopping When Tired or Stressed

    Both can lead to poorer decisions.

5. Stick to Perimeter Shopping

    The outer aisles typically house fresh produce, meats, and dairy.

6. Be Wary of Promotions

    Sales don't always align with your health goals—always check the product's nutritional quality.

This straightforward approach helps ensure your kitchen is stocked with nourishing foods, providing a solid foundation for healthier eating throughout the week.

KEEP A HEALTHY KITCHEN
AVOID STOCKING UNHEALTHY FOODS

Creating a supportive kitchen environment is one of the most impactful steps you can take toward maintaining long-term health and well-being. By designing your kitchen to prioritise nutritious choices and limit temptations, you make it easier to build consistent, healthy habits. This foundation not only helps you avoid impulsive decisions but also empowers you to stay aligned with your goals while enjoying a more balanced lifestyle.

Reduced Temptation

A kitchen free of unhealthy snacks and processed foods minimizes temptation, making it easier to stick to your health goals. When those items aren't easily accessible, you're less likely to indulge in impulsive or mindless eating.

A Healthier Household Environment

Creating a kitchen focused on nutritious options benefits everyone in your household. By reducing unhealthy temptations for the family, you foster a shared commitment to healthier habits and mutual support.

Encouragement of Better Habits

When nutritious options are prominently displayed, you naturally gravitate toward them. Fresh fruits on the counter or prepped vegetables at eye level in the fridge make healthier choices feel effortless. This setup reinforces positive habits and consistency.

Less Stress and More Enjoyment

An organised kitchen reduces the chaos of meal prep, making cooking more manageable and enjoyable. Knowing you have the tools and ingredients for a healthy meal removes the stress of last-minute decisions.

Support for Meal Planning

A kitchen stocked with the right staples makes meal planning and preparation easier. With essential ingredients readily available, you can try healthier recipes and avoid last-minute, less nutritious options.

Reduction in Food Waste

When your kitchen is well-organised, it's easier to use up ingredients before they spoil. Proper storage and planning mean fewer forgotten items in the back of the fridge and more efficient grocery use.

A Sense of Achievement

A supportive kitchen environment enhances your sense of control and achievement. Preparing balanced meals or reaching for nutritious snacks reinforces positive changes and builds motivation for success.

Strategies for Maintaining a Healthy Kitchen

1. Purge Unhealthy Items

    Remove snacks and drinks high in sugar, salt, or unhealthy fats from
    your kitchen. This limits temptation and promotes mindful choices.
    Donate unopened non-perishable items to a food bank to declutter
    while helping others.

2. Stock Up on Healthy Alternatives

    Replace unhealthy options with nutrient-rich choices like fruits, nuts,
    yogurt, and whole-grain snacks. Keeping a variety of healthy foods
    available ensures you always have satisfying options that prevent
    boredom.

3. Make Healthy Foods Visible

    Place fresh produce on counters or at eye level in the fridge to
    encourage better habits. When healthy foods are easy to see and reach,
    they become your first choice.

4. Adopt Smart Shopping Habits

    Use a grocery list focused on healthy items and plan meals for the week
    to avoid processed food aisles. Online shopping or curb-side pickup
    can reduce temptations and make the process more efficient.

5. Read Food Labels Carefully

    Pay attention to nutritional information, looking for hidden sugars and
    unhealthy fats. Avoid being swayed by misleading claims like "low-fat"
    or "natural," which can conceal unhealthy ingredients.

6. Prepare Meals in Advance

    Batch-cook healthy meals and store them for busy days to reduce
    reliance on takeout or processed foods. Prepping ahead ensures that
    nutritious options are always within reach.

7. Invest in Useful Kitchen Gadgets

   Blenders, steamers, and air fryers simplify the process of making healthy meals at home. These tools save time and make it easier to prepare nutrient-packed dishes.

8. Organise Your Kitchen

   Keep pantry staples and utensils tidy so you can quickly find what you need. An organised space streamlines meal prep and reduces frustration, helping you stay focused on healthier choices.

9. Limit Temptations

   If others in your household enjoy less healthy snacks, store them in a designated cupboard out of sight. This reduces the temptation to indulge while maintaining a supportive environment for your goals.

By tailoring your kitchen to support healthy eating, you set yourself up for consistent success. A thoughtfully maintained kitchen makes nutritious meals the default choice, reinforcing a balanced and fulfilling lifestyle.

FOCUS ON FIT, NOT WEIGHT
LET YOUR CLOTHES BE AN INDICATOR

Shifting attention from the number on the scale to how your clothes fit can be a more uplifting and comprehensive way to track progress. This perspective highlights total well-being and confidence, aligning perfectly with a lifestyle that values personal growth over purely numerical goals. Here's why this shift is so powerful:

Reflects Body Composition Changes

The scale doesn't differentiate between fat, muscle, or water weight, which can make it a poor tool for gauging overall progress. Muscle is denser than fat, so as you stay active and build muscle while losing fat, your weight may remain steady or even increase slightly. However, the fit of your clothes provides a more accurate and tangible reflection of these changes. Studies on body recomposition highlight how individuals focused on strength training often achieve better health outcomes despite minimal changes in weight. Looser clothing or improved muscle tone signals progress more meaningfully than a number on a scale.

Reduces Scale Anxiety

Frequent weigh-ins can lead to feelings of discouragement, as weight naturally fluctuates due to factors like water retention, hormone levels, and digestion. The psychological impact of these fluctuations can be significant, leading to frustration or even unhealthy behaviours like over-restricting food. Shifting the focus to how your clothes fit reduces this anxiety, allowing you to celebrate gradual, positive changes in how your body feels and functions instead of fixating on daily numbers.

Encourages a Positive Body Image

Focusing on how you feel in your clothes nurtures a more constructive self-perception. Research in psychology emphasises that body image is heavily influenced by how we interpret and evaluate our physical changes. By prioritising comfort, mobility, and capability over a specific weight, you foster a sense of self-worth that isn't tied to external validation. This mindset supports a healthier relationship with your body, enhancing both self-esteem and emotional resilience.

Provides a Motivation Boost

Nothing feels quite as rewarding as slipping into an old pair of jeans that didn't fit before. These non-scale victories provide tangible proof of progress and can be incredibly motivating. Psychologists explain that intrinsic motivators—such as the satisfaction of feeling stronger or healthier—are more sustainable than extrinsic ones like achieving a specific weight. By celebrating these milestones, you maintain enthusiasm for the habits that support your goals.

Aligns with Sustainable Lifestyle Changes

Focusing on how your clothes fit aligns with the idea of health as a long-term commitment rather than a short-term fix. Weight-centric goals can sometimes lead to yo-yo dieting, whereas paying attention to how you feel in your body fosters habits that are enjoyable and easier to maintain. This approach encourages a more relaxed and realistic attitude toward fitness and nutrition, making healthy living part of your daily routine.

Enhances Mindfulness and Self-Awareness

Paying attention to the fit of your clothes helps you tune into how your eating and exercise habits are impacting your body. This practice fosters mindfulness, encouraging you to reflect on what's working and where adjustments may be needed. Psychologists associate mindfulness with improved self-regulation, making it easier to make informed, intentional choices that align with your goals.

Reduces Obsession with Numbers

Constantly tracking weight can overshadow other valuable benefits of a healthy lifestyle, such as improved strength, endurance, and energy levels. Research into weight neutrality suggests that stepping away from numerical goals can reduce stress and create a more sustainable relationship with health. Shifting your focus to clothing fit allows you to appreciate the broader benefits of your efforts without being tied to the scale.

Supports Mental Well-being

By reducing the emphasis on weigh-ins, you alleviate the stress and frustration that often come with daily or weekly fluctuations. A positive, non-numerical focus encourages a healthier mindset, reducing feelings of defeat and promoting long-term success. Studies in behavioural psychology indicate that goals framed around capability and functionality—like fitting into comfortable clothing—are more likely to result in sustained behavioural change.

Practical Tips to Implement This Approach

1. Regularly Assess Fit

   Choose a specific outfit, such as a favourite pair of jeans or a fitted shirt, and try it on occasionally to track changes. Notice how it feels around key areas like your waist or shoulders to gauge progress in a simple, tangible way.

2. Set Non-Scale Goals

   Focus on goals that reflect your overall health, like building strength, improving endurance, or mastering a new skill. Achievements like running a little further or trying a challenging yoga pose provide clear markers of progress without relying on the scale.

3. Celebrate Non-Scale Victories

   Take note of improvements in areas like energy levels, mood, or sleep quality. These small milestones are meaningful signs of positive change and reinforce your efforts.

4. Avoid Frequent Weighing

   Consider reducing how often you weigh yourself or even putting the scale away. Shifting focus to how you feel and how your clothes fit reduces stress and encourages a more balanced approach to your health journey.

By focusing on clothing fit and non-scale victories, you create a healthier and more holistic approach to progress. This shift allows you to enjoy the journey, prioritising personal growth and long-term well-being over the pursuit of a specific number. Ultimately, the goal is to feel strong, capable, and content in your body. Letting your clothes guide your progress aligns with this vision, making the journey one of empowerment, confidence, and comprehensive wellness.

PRIORITISE SLEEP FOR WEIGHT LOSS, HEALTH, AND WELLBEING

Adequate sleep is a key but often overlooked aspect of a healthy lifestyle. Quality rest plays a fundamental role in weight management, overall health, and daily performance. Scientific research continues to highlight the profound impact of sleep on nearly every bodily system. Prioritising rest is not a luxury but an essential investment in your well-being.

Hormonal Balance

Sleep is a powerful regulator of the hormones ghrelin and leptin, which govern hunger and fullness. When sleep-deprived, ghrelin levels rise, intensifying hunger, while leptin levels drop, reducing your ability to feel satisfied. This imbalance often leads to overeating, particularly of high-calorie foods. Research shows that adequate sleep stabilises these hormones, helping to regulate appetite and avoid unnecessary calorie intake. Furthermore, sleep supports the regulation of cortisol, a stress hormone linked to abdominal fat storage, adding another layer of hormonal balance that aids weight management.

Metabolic Function

Your body's ability to metabolise carbohydrates and maintain stable blood sugar levels is closely tied to sleep. Sleep deprivation impairs insulin sensitivity, promoting fat storage and increasing the risk of metabolic disorders like diabetes. Chronic poor sleep disrupts your body's energy processing, making weight loss more difficult and fat gain more likely. However, adequate sleep enhances metabolic function, improving glucose regulation and enabling the body to burn fat more efficiently. Additionally, well-rested individuals tend to have more consistent energy levels, making them better equipped to maintain an active lifestyle, which further supports weight management.

Reduced Cravings

Fatigue significantly increases cravings for sugary or high-carbohydrate foods as your body seeks quick energy fixes. At the same time, sleep deprivation reduces impulse control, making it harder to resist unhealthy options. Studies confirm that sleep-deprived individuals are more likely to snack unnecessarily and consume extra calories. Quality sleep curbs these cravings, allowing for better food choices and improved dietary consistency. Sleep also optimises your brain's reward system, helping you feel more satisfied with healthier meals, which reduces the temptation to indulge in calorie-dense snacks.

Emotional and Mental Health

Sleep is integral to managing stress and emotional well-being. Chronic sleep deprivation heightens stress hormone levels, such as cortisol, which can lead to overeating and fat storage. Lack of sleep also contributes to mood swings, irritability, and reduced motivation, all of which can undermine efforts to maintain healthy habits. In contrast, a well-rested mind is more resilient, better equipped to handle daily stressors, and less likely to rely on food for emotional comfort. Sleep also enhances focus and emotional stability, enabling you to stay consistent with long-term health and weight goals.

Physical Performance

Sleep is essential for recovery and optimal physical performance, which are crucial for weight management and overall health. During sleep, your body repairs muscle tissue, synthesises proteins, and releases growth hormones necessary for fat metabolism and muscle maintenance. Individuals who prioritise sleep report greater endurance, better coordination, and higher performance during physical activities. Furthermore, well-rested individuals tend to engage more effectively in exercise routines, burning more calories and achieving better results. Sleep also helps prevent the fatigue that can lead to exercise-related injuries, ensuring that physical activity remains a sustainable part of your lifestyle.

Injury Prevention

Inadequate sleep impairs coordination, reaction times, and balance, significantly increasing the likelihood of injuries. Whether exercising, driving, or completing daily tasks, being well-rested improves alertness and reduces accident risk. Studies consistently show that individuals who get sufficient sleep are less likely to experience workplace or fitness-related injuries. By preventing setbacks caused by fatigue, adequate sleep ensures you can maintain an active lifestyle, which supports both weight and overall health.

Energy Balance

Sleep is critical for restoring energy and maintaining balance, both physically and mentally. Without enough rest, you may experience midday fatigue and an increased reliance on sugary or high-calorie snacks for a quick energy boost. Over time, this cycle can disrupt healthy eating habits and lead to weight gain. Quality sleep replenishes your energy stores, ensuring you wake up refreshed and capable of sustaining an active, productive lifestyle. This stable energy balance supports healthier dietary choices and promotes the consistency needed for long-term weight management.

Tips for Improving Sleep

1. Establish a Consistent Schedule

    Go to bed and wake at the same time daily.

2. Create a Sleep-Friendly Environment

    Keep your bedroom dark, quiet, and cool.

3. Limit Screen Exposure Before Bed

    Blue light disrupts melatonin production.

4. Watch Caffeine and Alcohol Intake

    Both can interfere with restful sleep.

5. Develop a Relaxing Bedtime Routine

    Gentle activities like reading or stretching signal your body to wind down.

6. Stay Active During the Day

    Regular exercise promotes deeper, more restful sleep.

7. Mind Your Diet

    Heavy or spicy meals late in the evening can disrupt sleep.

Prioritising sleep is one of the most impactful steps you can take for your health and well-being. A good night's rest doesn't just leave you feeling refreshed—it optimises your physical, mental, and emotional readiness for each day. By cultivating healthy sleep habits, you equip yourself to approach life with clarity, energy, and enthusiasm. Sleep isn't a luxury; it's a foundation for living a balanced and fulfilling life. Make it a priority, and the benefits will ripple across every aspect of your health and happiness.

INVEST IN A HEALTHY COOKBOOK: QUICK, HEALTHY MEALS MADE EASY

A cookbook focused on quick, healthy recipes is a valuable resource, especially if you're juggling a busy schedule. It provides both inspiration and practical guidance. Here's how a healthy cookbook can elevate your meal planning:

Variety of options

A good cookbook includes recipes for all meal times—breakfast, lunch, dinner, and snacks—ensuring your diet remains varied and exciting. Exploring different cuisines and flavours broadens your skills and keeps meals interesting.

Time-saving recipes

Many cookbooks focus on quick meals you can prepare in 30 minutes or less, helping you enjoy nutritious, home-cooked dishes without spending hours in the kitchen.

Nutritional information

Health-focused cookbooks often include detailed information about calories, macronutrients, and micronutrients. This helps you align meals with your specific dietary goals or nutritional needs.

Cooking tips and techniques

Beyond recipes, cookbooks provide practical advice for efficient chopping, seasoning, and cooking methods that preserve nutrients. Learning these skills refines your home-cooking abilities and builds confidence in adapting recipes.

Inspiration for healthy eating

An engaging cookbook motivates you to try new dishes, making mealtime enjoyable rather than a chore. This variety prevents boredom and keeps you from returning to less nutritious eating habits.

Meal planning help

Some cookbooks offer structured meal plans, which simplify grocery shopping, reduce food waste, and keep your week's meals organised and balanced.

Alignment with dietary needs

The right cookbook matches your dietary preferences, such as vegetarian, vegan, gluten-free, or low-carb. This alignment helps you stick to your plan while ensuring meals remain enjoyable and satisfying.

What to look for in a Healthy Cookbook

1. Recipes for all meal times to keep your diet varied.

2. Quick, time-saving recipes with clear instructions.

3. Nutritional details to help you make informed choices.

4. Practical tips for cooking efficiently and preserving nutrients.

5. Creative ingredient swaps to make meals healthier.

6. Structured meal plans to simplify shopping and preparation.

7. Alignment with your specific dietary preferences or restrictions.

A healthy cookbook can be a game-changer in your journey towards weight loss and balanced living. It's more than just a collection of recipes; it's a tool that inspires creativity in the kitchen, encourages better food choices, and simplifies meal planning. By incorporating quick, delicious, and nutritious meals into your routine, you'll find it easier to stay on track without feeling deprived. Whether you're new to cooking or an experienced home chef, the right cookbook can provide fresh ideas and practical solutions to support your weight loss goals and transform your relationship with food. Invest in one today and take a step closer to a healthier, more fulfilling lifestyle.

Books to Consider

1. The Skinnytaste Cookbook by Gina Homolka

    Offers light, flavourful dishes that are easy to prepare, with nutritional information for every recipe.

2. Fit Men Cook by Kevin Curry

    Features simple, healthy recipes designed for busy lifestyles, with an emphasis on meal prep and balanced eating.

3. Quick & Easy Meals: Delicious Healthy Recipes in Under 30 Minutes by Joe Wicks

    Focuses on nutritious meals that can be prepared quickly, ideal for people on tight schedules.

4. Minimalist Baker's Everyday Cooking by Dana Shultz

    A collection of simple recipes requiring 10 ingredients or less, designed to be healthy and quick to make.

5. Healthy Meal Prep Cookbook by Toby Amidor

    Includes meal prep-friendly recipes that are both nutritious and easy to make ahead of time.

6. Half Baked Harvest Super Simple by Tieghan Gerard

    Offers a variety of wholesome, easy-to-follow recipes with a focus on fresh ingredients.

7. The Clean Plate: Eat, Reset, Heal by Gwyneth Paltrow

    Includes healthy recipes designed for quick preparation, focusing on clean eating and whole foods.

EMBARK ON YOUR GREATEST JOURNEY

As you turn the final page of Weight Loss Without Dieting, remember that this book is more than a guide; it's the beginning of a profound transformation. It's about reclaiming control over your health and discovering a sustainable, fulfilling way of living—free from the restrictive cycles of dieting. This journey is not about deprivation but about empowerment, balance, and creating a lifestyle that truly works for you.

The path you've explored in these chapters is just the starting point. Ahead lies a life brimming with energy, confidence, and the freedom to embrace all the opportunities that come with a healthier you. Each strategy and insight you've gained is a tool, a compass to guide you as you make choices that reflect your goals and values. This is a personal expedition that continues far beyond the pages of this book, shaping not only your weight but also your overall sense of vitality and purpose.

Every small step matters. Whether it's incorporating mindful eating, embracing movement you enjoy, or making time to recharge, each decision builds toward a stronger, more capable version of yourself. This isn't just about weight loss; it's about creating a lifestyle that fosters growth, resilience, and joy. The benefits you'll experience—more energy, enhanced confidence, and better health—will ripple across every aspect of your life, enriching your relationships, career, and passions.

This journey doesn't end here. It evolves with you, as each new habit and milestone adds momentum to your progress. Let every choice you make reflect your commitment to living boldly and authentically. The challenges you face will only reinforce your determination, showing you just how much you're capable of achieving.

Stay curious and open to learning. Embrace this process as an ongoing opportunity for growth, self-discovery, and empowerment. Surround yourself with experiences, people, and goals that inspire and motivate you. Celebrate your progress, no matter how small, and remember that every positive decision brings you closer to the life you've envisioned.

Your journey is waiting, filled with endless possibilities and untapped potential. Step forward with confidence, knowing you have the tools and knowledge to thrive. This is your time to build a life defined not by restrictions but by the freedom to live healthily and happily on your terms. Embrace each day as a chance to grow, to shine, and to celebrate all that you are becoming. The future is yours—live it fully, with purpose and joy.

Printed in Dunstable, United Kingdom